GYM JUNKIES

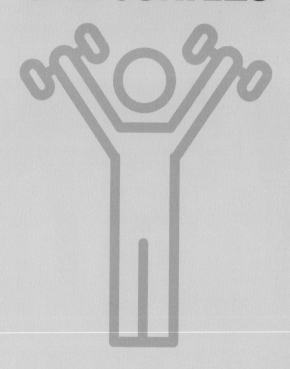

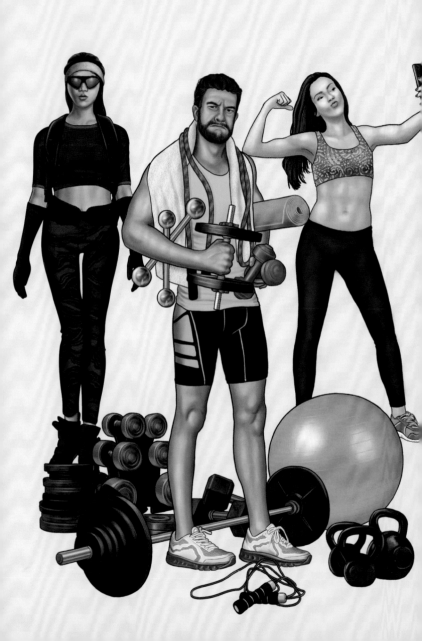

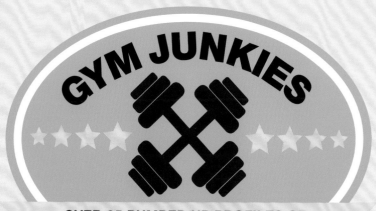

GYM JUNKIES

OVER 25 PUMPED-UP PROFILES OF GYM BUNNIES AND FITNESS FREAKS

SIMON GLAZIN

DOG 'n' BONE

Published in 2018 by Dog 'n' Bone Books
An imprint of Ryland Peters & Small Ltd

20–21 Jockey's Fields   341 E 116th St
London WC1R 4BW   New York, NY 10029

www.rylandpeters.com

10 9 8 7 6 5 4 3 2 1

A CIP catalog record for this book is available from
the Library of Congress and the British Library.

ISBN: 978 1 911026 50 1

Printed in China

Editor: Dawn Bates
Designer: Jerry Goldie
Illustrator: Paul Parker
Icon illustrations from Flaticon.
All icons designed by Freepik
except for the following:
Smashicons p5 top, p8, p10
top; Becris p5, fouth from top;
Dave Gandy p16; Made by
Made p24; Prosymbols p48;
Turkkub p58.

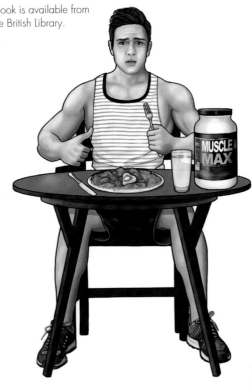

CONTENTS

INTRODUCTION

According to statistics, there are nearly 132 million gym memberships worldwide. And apparently that amounts to an industry worth approximately $76 billion. To put that figure into perspective, it just beats Mark Zuckerberg's net worth. And guess what? We probably spend just as much time a year on Facebook as we do working out. In fact, the number of people using Facebook whilst peddling furiously on the exercise bike must be huge! Surely gyms can now be considered a social network all of their own?

Whether it's to let off pent up steam from an infuriating boss, escape a nagging spouse, spy on your crush, show off your new "gear," or, erm, oh yeah… to shift some pounds and/or tone up, going to the gym has now become as important as brushing your teeth, getting dressed, or putting on deodorant. (Hell, we wish more people would put on deodorant in the gym!)

Despite the increase in the number of memberships, there still must be lots of us who spend more of our time at the gym people watching than, you know, actually working out. Side-eyeing that guy who spends a little too long staring at his reflection while simultaneously chest pressing, or laughing under your breath at The Prehistoric Noise Makers is much more fun than working up a sweat on the cross-trainer. If only someone would note down these observations of all the preeners and posers. What a brilliant book that would make! Oh wait...

You're about to meet a lot of very familiar faces from your time at the gym: some you love, some you loathe, and a few you can probably personally relate to. There'll be some "uh huh!" moments, and you might even realize you are one of these personalities. That's OK though. We won't tell anyone.

Happy workouts, everyone!

THE BROMANCERS

Among the new Gen Z buzzwords that have made it into the dictionary—dabbing, airplane mode, cheat days—there's bromance. Thanks, not least, to countless reality TV shows, heterosexual male friends can now get away with walking down the street cuddling, drunk kissing, and escorting each other to the bathroom. And now gyms across the country are spawning all-new bromances to rival those in any club, bar, or on TV. Have you spotted any of these bromancers at yours?

THOSE THAT SPUR
Usually found in a pack of three, these are among the loudest in the gym habitat. Two shout words of encouragement and profanities, while the other busts a gut pushing much more weight than he should. The process is repeated until all three are red-faced and sweaty. Then onto the next machine or exercise for more of the same

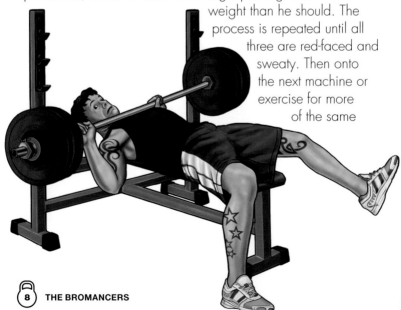

boyish plaudits. The usual mating calls include backslapping, whooping, and, rarely, and quite unsightly, one being picked up in some kind of victory dance.

THOSE THAT OVER-SHARE

Crowding round their prey—in this case the carcass of a punching bag—these bromancers regale each other with their carnal conquests. Don't get too close, though… you might overhear something that will disturb you for the rest of your workout, possibly your life. This species is up for anything. In special cases, they might even whip out their phones to show off their latest conquest. Intrigued, you'll want to look, and by all means do if you can get away with it. But be warned, you'll get hooked on their soap-drama sex lives. An interesting way of keeping you coming back to the gym, though.

THOSE THAT SPOT

Ever seen one guy standing over another doing chest presses? No, they're not in the middle of a wild argument. No, he hasn't got him pinned to the bench. He is spotting him, or to the rest of us, making sure he doesn't decapitate himself with one too many reps with the barbell. To "spot" is to help. If you see your "other half" struggle to lift that weight, you step in with words of encouragement and sometimes a gentle push in the right direction. Usually just shadowing his arm movements is enough—he won't actually drop the weights—well, you hope not. You don't want to be that spotter who looked the other way for one too many seconds.

THE NEW YEAR'S RESOLUTIONERS

New year, new you. If you have to read this annoying, passive-aggressive catchphrase one more time... But come January 3rd (we all know New Year's resolutions don't start until the 3rd; the 1st and 2nd are still "hangover" days), you know you'll have a brand-new membership for the gym, ready to work off those extra pounds collected during the festivities. So how do you spot someone who has put "get fit" at the top of their list?

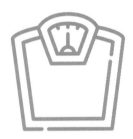

The NY Resolutioner will walk into the gym, all fresh-faced and ready to go. They'll be in brand-new "gym gear" that was on their Christmas list—so new in fact that the fresh-out-of-the-online-packaging fold lines are still visible. They'll have shiny new earphones and never-worn-before sneakers. They'll stand at the front of the gym for a good few minutes, assessing what machine to approach first. No one will acknowledge them because no one will have seen them before. As they mount the cross-trainer with trepidation in their eyes, they'll spend the next five minutes trying desperately to work out how to turn the thing on, only to realize, eventually, that you actually have to start moving your legs for the LED display to ping into action. They will spend as long as they can on there, breaking out into a sweat on

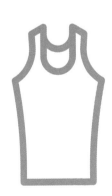

minute seven or eight, and stopping for a breather on minute 13. They'll think it's the hardest thing they've ever done, possibly comparing it to climbing Everest, and by minute 21 they'll be off the machine and lying on their back on a mat trying to catch their breath, while attempting what might 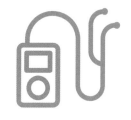 possibly resemble a sit-up to a trained eye, but looks more like a beached whale side shuffle to everyone else.

They'll feel really pleased with themselves, and so they should. To pull yourself away from the chocolate bowl and nearly stale mince pies is an achievement. You'll see them back again the day after, and the day after that. You'll even catch a glimpse of them a handful of times during the second and third weeks of January. They will more than likely be churning out the same routine every single time. But that's OK. They're building stamina.

By week four, you'll notice their commitment dwindle. By the middle of February, you'll spot them maybe once a week. March will be a no-show altogether. In April they'll remember they joined three months ago and are still paying for membership, so turn up a couple of times, and by May… you can work it out.

You'll see them in July again, though, for two weeks solid, then in August with a deep golden tan once or twice. Then never again. They are very much the enigma of the gym world.

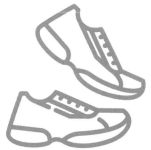

THE BODY BUILDER 2.0

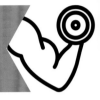

You think you've seen it all until you spot Mr Body Builder 2.0 in the gym car park, downing his concoction of five eggs and whey protein, pre- and post-workout. While you try to hold back the sick just thinking about it, he's on his fourth round of protein super-smoothies of the day. God only knows what would happen if he misses one... he'd deflate maybe?

Once inside the gym, he's all pufferfish cheeks and snakelike veins as he does rep after rep of bicep curls with the 50kg weights. The only contact you've had with these dumbbells is stubbing your toe, and styling it out as a burpee. Just when you think his arms might pop, he moves on to weighted squats to further sculpt his legs and bum. Not that his legs need any more help... they resemble the hilliest of countryside terrain already.

And while most of us have learnt to waist belt thanks to TV stylists' incessant chat about how it gives you such a fabulous shape, these guys belt up in case their torsos decide to suddenly fold in on themselves or their backs just give up all together. A harder-working accessory you're yet to meet.

Look carefully, and you're likely to spot The Body Builder's sidekick, usually standing in the wings, ready to rescue him should his shoulders stop working. The Sidekick is almost always at least the equivalent of two dress sizes smaller. Think of him as the student. You might even hear the odd "whoop" of encouragement or cheer from the sidelines after the beefcake completes another successful rep of curls.

With his sights firmly set on being an Arnold Schwarzenegger size, Body Builder 2.0 crashes his way round the gym, Neanderthal-like, shoulder-pressing whatever he can find en route to the weights rack, while all the other puny men just watch on in awe. One day, one day soon.

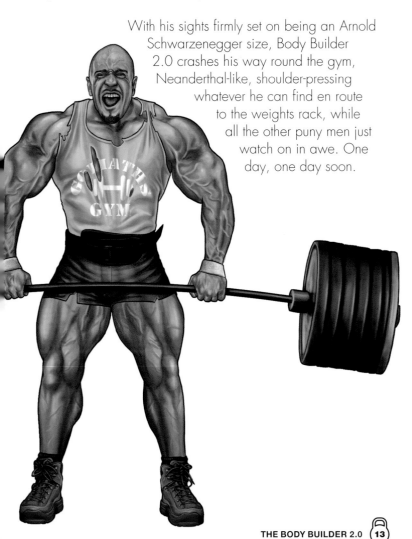

COUPLES WHO GYM TOGETHER

While single millennials are still aggressively swiping right, hoping that Mr or Mrs Right Now pops up next, the lucky few who have found "the one" are happily parading them round the gym in full view, sometimes even fitting in PDAs that are, quite frankly, unforgivable. As our working hours get longer and longer, the only way to make time for the significant other is to invite him or her to places you never thought you would. Plus-ones are usually reserved for swanky after-work events and charity galas, not 45 minutes on the running machine. And for those of us who must endure your need to kiss after every sit-up, why not do us all a favor and find the most remote corner of the gym? Or maybe just keep it at home? Novel, I know.

You see, you put yourself in a Catch-22 position: to the single people, those who struggle to get a slot with the personal trainer, let alone a date, you'll always be that couple who hold hands on the rowing machine. They end up despising you for being so happy—loathing you for bringing your perfect relationship into the one place they don't have to think about going home to a microwave meal for one.

To some of the people coupled up, you represent everything their relationship is not. They may well have escaped to the gym after an explosive argument at home, only to be faced with the both of you staring lovingly into each other's eyes, undressing each other during the last round of kettlebell swings. What they definitely do not want to see is you two, fornicating over the free weights. Why do you think they row harder, punch faster, or step quicker when you both walk past? To release the anger, that's why.

But, and get ready for a moment of true honesty, to the masses you are just annoying. Two friends spurring each other on with a backslap is fine, or a personal trainer resting on your pelvic bone to release years of pent-up stretching is perfectly acceptable. But pure, unadulterated PDAs are just so beyond what most people sign up for.

Smooching, holding hands, high-fiving, none of these things are OK between two people in love, at the gym.

You can't win with this one. No ifs. No buts. There's a reason why the "joint membership" box is seldom ticked on sign-up… most people use their gym time as "me time," meaning partners are most definitely not invited. And you never hear any gym staff offer the "married special" membership, because they are au fait with what can happen should an ex waltz through the door, or if there's a spousal disagreement during a spin class. It ain't pretty.

THE TEACHER'S PET

You're one step away from bringing the instructor an apple, such is your enthusiasm for classes. You thank God every day that your gym is open 24 hours and has a personal trainer willing to do a midnight stretching class. You can't handle not having a routine, so much so that your iPhone diary is full of color-coded dots to indicate: spin classes (green), pump (red), Absolutely Abs (orange), and yoga (Downward Dog Purple—the new Pantone color for this year maybe?). You can quite happily class-hop, and have managed three in a row with a break for a protein energy ball. You know every instructor by name, and they you, so when stand-ins turn up you're completely put out that they don't give you special treatment. You know most of the routines by heart, and are usually that annoying person at the front almost one step ahead of the teacher. You even join in with that real Americanism of clapping and whooping when the class ends. It's easy to spot which class you're most obsessed with…

CAUTION

WET FLOOR

SPINNING

You're wearing those weird, grown-up nappy Lycra shorts with the padding that protects the "gooch" (that bit between your… oh whatever!). You've also got the shoes that clip in to the pedals to avoid feet slippage, usually practiced by the rest of us. Be careful as you run to grab the bike closest to teacher. Those shoes have no grip and you don't want to stack it in front of your hero, do you?

BODYPUMP

Woe betide anyone that takes your rightful spot on the classroom floor, or the last 5kg weight for that matter. Getting on the list for a Bodypump class is harder than putting your name down for a Birkin bag, hence why most people come out, head down on their phones, furiously trying to book next week's session.

YOGA

Even though mats are provided, you carry your orange one round with you everywhere, like some kind of Dior accessory. "I just prefer mine." Without even knowing what class you've just come out of, your complete state of Zen gives the game away.

STEP

Not content with being about to hike the equivalent of 45 floors, your warm-up is using the step machine three minutes before, just to get your thighs used to the burn. If you lurk outside a studio before a step class, you'll spot mostly middle-aged women who look set to conquer Everest. For the over-60s, it's escalators.

AB FAB ABS

For every three people who finish an abs class, there's one holding their abdomen in agony. Either they think that one 22-minute class (eight minutes is taken up by stretching and moaning) will result in a six-pack, or they've never used a single stomach muscle in their life, other than the ones that get them out of bed in the morning.

MOMS
ON THE RUN

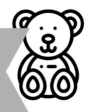

Why they haven't invented a treadmill with a baby seat attached to it is beyond The Busy Moms©. If supermarkets can do it with their trolleys, why can't the running machine brands? Even though the majority of their gym visits are to escape motherhood, it's sometimes easier to have Baby next to you to avoid the incessant WhatsApp messages from the Father Who Knows Nothing or the Babysitter Who Can't Control. There are, however, a few different species of The Busy Mom©. Spotted any of these?

THE DETERMINED
This set refuse to let gravity take its course. Mother Nature will not define their procreational rights with any form of sagging skin or leftover bump. These mothers want their prechild bodies back, and they're doing everything possible to achieve it. Personal trainers, 300 mountain climbers, 15 minutes on the battle ropes (if you know, you know!). These women will happily chuck little Billy or cute Megan into the crèche downstairs for 10 minutes of unadulterated, uninterrupted, repetitive pelvic floor exercises, because they definitely will NOT be that mother wetting themselves when they sneeze at the school gates.

THE GOSSIPERS
We've all seen and heard them. A few friends, sitting legs akimbo on the mats, nattering away, thinking they are doing the world of good to their hamstrings, when in actual fact they are just pissing off their neighbor who is trying to hold the plank for longer than a minute. "I just couldn't believe it!

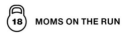

She turned up wearing that dress again. It was awful the first time!" or "Apparently they're divorcing, but listen, I don't know for sure so don't say anything," or even: "Oh I know, their son is such a little ＊＊＊＊, I don't know how they cope!" What's that phrase…? If you haven't got anything nice to say, get the hell out of the gym? These mothers categorically did not sign up to the gym to tone up or slim down. They are purely there for the smoke and mirrors, to let people believe they are actually working out.

THE SCHOOL MOMS

This fashion-savvy bunch have the latest Stella McCartney Adidas gear on and the best sneakers money, or their husband's, can buy. They do the school drop-off in their athleisure, jogging on the spot, sending smiley Jasmine off through the playground. Then off they sprint to their 4x4, and into the gym they go. Statistically* 50 percent don't make it through the gym doors. They don't even make it to the gym car park. They don't even make it to the same road/area/town as the gym. They detour to the shopping mall where racking up their step count is the only form of cardio for the day. The other 50 percent stay true to their school-gate amateur dramatic performance. They complete their circuits, or the Bums, Tums, and Thighs class, and even post about it on social media, because if it's not on Facebook, it didn't actually happen.

*Not official

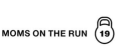

THE BEACH BOYS (AND GIRLS)

Consider, for a minute, ever feeling brave enough (or, in fact, ever feeling the need) to work out in next to nothing, in full view of, well, everyone, in the blazing sunshine, with plenty of onlookers taking selfies in disbelief. I know, it's a ludicrous, preposterous idea, isn't it? Hands up who just fancies going completely unnoticed during their workout instead? But in some far-reaching climes, places where the mystical "sun" does actually put his hat on, there are folk that bear all and flex their biceps, where people go to press-up for attention and to top up their tan. Yes, the beach gym is a thing.

It'd be safe to say that 99 percent of beach regulars congregate on the good old sand for three things: vitamin D, frozen margaritas, and to read whatever is on the current book club list. You get comfy, and when no one is looking, whip off your top or bikini cover-up and lay horizontal for the foreseeable. You only ever get up to take a drink from someone or to throw yourself in the sea to cool down. To sit up would be to expose your usually neatly concealed rolls (yes, even the thinnest of us have at least one roll when sitting up!).

The 1 percent are those people that are so confident, so cocksure, so in desperate need of attention (we're just jealous really) that they take a break from basting themselves to drop and do 50. These gym junkies are so serious about raising their heart rates and pumping iron that they can't even wait to do the "too-hot sand dance" to take it inside. They rival those that don't even make it out the gym door before devouring a can of tuna to keep protein levels to a maximum. Don't expect to see "ordinary" people lifting the dumbbells either. Oh no. These ones are reserved for mostly topless men, in the shortest of short shorts, sporting either a top knot or shiny bald head, called Hank or Titan.

While some of you might think Muscle Beach is just a fictional place full of meatheads and women body builders, it is, in fact, a real place full of meatheads and women body builders. The beach gyms of the east coast of America are visible from space, thanks to the heat coming off those working out—both in temperature and looks. They are the equivalent of human aquariums… premium viewing times are pre-8am and post-real life. Outdoor gyms are now popping up in towns all around the UK too. Granted, they are government-funded, look a bit naff, and usually attract the local yobs, but Arnold Schwarzenegger had to start somewhere.

THE OAPS
(OLD AGE PUSH-UPS)

There are only two types of people at the gym at 6am: the Pre-Work Keenos—those who have an important breakfast meeting, but need some adrenaline to get through it—and The Oldies—those who have already been awake for three hours because of excess flatulence and have sucked their dentures in from the glass beside their bed. Whatever your personal opinions are of the maximum age limit to operate the spin bike, you've got to give it to the OAPs... their sheer stamina to get up every single morning and do the same routine is quite remarkable.

Pre-World War II Albert's daily circuit of 10 minutes on the treadmill (speed: snail), 10 sets of bicep curls (weight: his walking stick), and a couple of goes on the kettlebells is as important as his free over-60s daily coffee from the local café. It keeps him motivated to haul himself out of bed every morning.

And for Doris, who doesn't mind telling anyone who asks, and even those who haven't so much as looked at her, that she is "older than water and can still lift her leg over her head," it's her chance to pull herself away from all that dreary morning television, playing bridge, and baking and to have a little chat with… well, anyone who'll listen. She's not fussy.

There are some gyms that offer an "OAP hour," which usually involves little working out and more shuffling from one machine to the next, but let's face it, give them 20 minutes and they'll be back in their mobility scooter faster than you can say "pass the prune juice." You'll know when you've accidentally stumbled upon OAP hour… you'll just know.

If you are at your local place of workout worship while an OAP is present, there are a few things to be aware of:

- Deadlifts could be just that—deadly. If they're struggling with that barbell, go give them a hand.
- One wrong move on a treadmill and it's pensioner DOWN. Be on the lookout.
- The leg press machine is a quick way to a hip break. Don't leave them unattended.
- If you've spotted an oldie in the gym, be mindful of not leaving a medicine ball in the middle of the floor—without their bifocals on, it's a hazard waiting to happen.
- If they look like they've stopped breathing halfway through stretching their 80-year-old hamstrings, they probably have. Either that or they've just fallen asleep. A little prod can determine either way.

THE ALL-MADE-UP GIRLS

Now that basically anyone can add MUA (makeup artist) to the end of their Instagram handle and believe their own lies, and thanks to the Kardashians ever-important introduction of contouring (honestly, what did we do before face sculpting?), more and more women are heading out to the gym in a full face of slap. They can obviously do what they like, when they like, but it does beg the question... WTF?

A night on the tiles, a posh dinner, a first date, a big party, even a day in the office—all events that for sure require a slick of makeup (or a full face, whatever your preference). And even though you might get hot and sweaty in your favorite club, you can reapply as and when you see fit. However, having a full face of makeup sliding down your face because you've spent one too many minutes on the cross-trainer is really not the one.

There are usually a few reasons why you'd turn up to the gym with a full face on:

1. You really couldn't care less what other people think. You wear makeup everywhere but in bed, except when you're too drunk to take it off.
2. You're a bride-to-be and have just had a makeup trial. You had 45 seconds to spare until the uber strict Body Pump teacher closed the doors and denied anyone else entry.
3. You're a model and have come straight from a photoshoot with no time to spare to remove it. Yes, the shoot brief just read: DRAG QUEEN.

4. You are a drag queen.
5. You are on the "walk of shame" home and decided to nip in for a quick half an hour on the rowing machine to sweat out all the shots you sunk before going home with… what was his name again?

There are obvious times when applying a thin layer of waterproof mascara, a little eye pencil, and some blusher is absolutely fine though:

1. There's a cute boy you spotted a couple of days ago, and even though you don't mind him seeing you in your Lycra, you want to look like you've made a bit of an effort. He doesn't need to see what you look like first thing in the morning, fresh-faced, just yet.
2. You've come straight from the office, and whereas usually you'd have time to take off your makeup with a wipe before heading to the gym, your last meeting with Gary from accounts ran over.
3. You've heard that Dolly Parton sleeps in a full face just in case there's a fire and she needs to be evacuated from her building. You don't want to face a gang of firefighters with not a scrap on!

THE HOARD WORKER

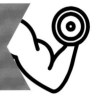

You can tell a lot about a person from how they behave at the gym. You know the heavy grunters are going to be loudmouths, those who nearly kill themselves doing sit-ups are determined at life, the people who flit from machine to machine after 2.5 minutes on each are not to be trusted, and those that hoard equipment are beyond selfish. The truth is, sex noises are easily overcome with headphones turned up to the max, determined individuals are to be praised, and those who can't commit are still probably lovely to talk to. But the selfish hoarders… they are a liability, a law unto themselves, irrational, irresponsible, incompetent, and all the other hateful adjectives that start with an "i."

Picture the scene (and try not to get angry): you've done your 30 minutes' hard slog on the bike, you've completed 45 minutes on level eight on the cross-trainer's "Fat Burn" option, you've reached your goal of 2,500 miles rowed, you've successfully shoulder-pressed the equivalent of 12 fully grown male Golden Retrievers and, now, just when you thought you couldn't sweat anymore, it's time for those all-important bicep curls. (You've heard the personal trainer's fool-proof routine to a regular, and made a mental note of how to get "the big guns," as he put it. You feel proud that you've saved the $100 per hour fee.)

You lock eyes with the weight rack. You pad over, cautiously, like a tiger hunting its prey. You scan those cold steel shelves up and down as you get nearer to locate what you are looking for. To your utter horror the weights you need aren't there. You start to panic. You frantically swing round to face the benches to see if anyone is using them—you'll sit patiently if they are. No one has them. Then you notice that the weights that usually sit either side of yours haven't been put back either. And no one at the benches has them. It twigs. There's a hoarder among you.

Off you huff around the floor, in a rage that someone would be so selfish, so mindless to dare to use your intended dumbbells without putting them back. As you approach the mats, that one area usually reserved for stretching and cooling down, you spot the culprit. There they are, in all their greedy, self-centered glory, completely surrounded by various gym accoutrements— barbells, dumbbells, skipping ropes, kettlebells—when all they are doing is tying themselves up like a pretzel to stretch their hamstrings. Livid is an understatement. If this real-life situation were a cartoon sketch, you'd be that character with steam spouting from your ears.

"Are you using that?" You ask with full force, almost barking it at the miscreant. And when they calmly reply with: "Oh no, I'm done with all of this", you have to mentally count to five and try your damnedest not to wrap the nearest barbell around their neck.

Off you stomp, with the prized weights in tow, ready to start the routine you so expertly nicked from the personal trainer, only to find there isn't one single bench available to use. You admit defeat, and take yourself off for a McFlurry, cursing all the way.

THE HEART-THROB

Remember the cult '90s board game Dream Phone? Pulling out a card at random, dialing that generic phone number on the pink phone, and hearing the clues from the dreamboat on the other end. The idea was to find out who had a crush on you—Mike, Dave, Gary… hardly exotic names, but there was something about those floppy-haired hunks. Every gym has a Dream Phone boy or two, and although they might be slightly more cryptic than their cardboard counterparts, they are there to be marveled at and swooned over.

Yes, we all have different tastes, but The Heart-throb transcends good looks. You might like short, bald men in real life, but your fantasy man—the one all women and gay man have tucked away in their minds—has just walked into the gym. Just like Barbie's Ken is hot because, well, he's hot, this guy is drop-dead gorgeous personified. But there are two clear types of The Heart-throb. Which one are you, and/or which do you prefer?

THE ONE WHO KNOWS HE'S HOT
This guy has the swagger of Justin Timberlake, the looks of Zac Efron, but the attitude of Justin Bieber. He knows he's hot, and that's just annoying. You don't want to fancy him, you try your best not to look in his direction, but you can't help yourself. He'll go out of his way to make it known he has arrived: laughing a little too loudly, pushing weights a little too enthusiastically, and shaking his protein shake a little too provocatively. He knows everyone in the gym, no matter what time it

is. Or maybe this Mr Arrogant just thinks he knows everyone and everyone should know him. He comes to work out and to be seen in equal measure, possibly the latter a little bit more.

THE ONE WHO KNOWS HE'S HOT, BUT PLAYS IT DOWN

You'll never know that he's actually at the gym until you spot him. He's the stealth heart-throb, and even though he knows he has the looks, he's very happy to go under the radar. This automatically makes him more attractive than Mr Arrogant. To look smoking and sweaty is an art form, and he has nailed it. This is the guy that you'll happily, and discreetly, move your stretching mat for to parts of the gym you never knew existed, just to catch a glimpse of his ass in those shorts. You've even hopped onto a machine you've never used before just to be next to him for the two minutes you survived not knowing what the hell you are doing. To fall flat on your face right now might be a disaster or a bonus: he might finally take notice of you. You've held eye contact before, a pivotal moment in your gym career, which instantly makes you feel like a 13-year-old kid again, playing Dream Phone with your friends.

Whichever you chose from the above, make sure to never share with anyone that you secretly know The Heart-throb's gym schedule and that you plan your trips around his. It sounds just as weird now you've read it on this page as it does out loud.

THE FASHION NAYSAYERS

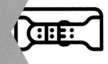

Sartorial choices should not matter at the gym. But they do. A lot. If you think it's a safe place devoid of judgment and whispered insults, you're so wrong. The gym is now akin to a fashion show, with the editors-in-chief (best dressed) pursing lips at bad decisions and bloggers (fashion-forward dressers) taking selfies.

There are other priorities, we get it—perfecting the plank, progressing to heavier weights, shifting the pounds with cardio. But you don't want to be called out for turning up looking like a dog's dinner. Or worse… in last season's leggings. You can guarantee your gym has a blog that picks the best and worst gym looks, written anonymously by the receptionist who takes sneaky pictures as you walk through the door. You don't want to end up on that, so pick the category that best describes your gym style, and choose one you want to be a member of instead…

THE FASHION-FORWARD THINKERS (FFT)

You knew you'd recognized that jeweled Lycra top; it was star buy in the new Vogue. And "Why do her leggings look brand new and mine look like they've been dragged through a hedge?" Because they are fresh out the packet! The FFT woman isn't scared of clashing prints and colors, which annoys everyone else because it all looks brilliant together. And FFT man wears mottled gray shorts over black "meggings" with such confidence that five more turn up the next day in the same combination.

THE CHUCK-ON-AND-GOERS

You spot the gym gear on the floor that you wore two days previous, sniff it to make sure it's wearable, and pull it on. The first T-shirt you find will do, and the only sneakers by the front door are the ones you walk the dog in. It's not until you see your reflection in the gym studio that you realize you look like the laundry has exploded all over you. It's OK, though, you'll go out of your way not to say hello to anyone you know—just plug your headphones in and keep the world out.

THE TOO-TIGHT BRIGADE

We're all for super-stretch, man-made fabrics (hello, Spanks!), but there are limits. This is mainly for the men. Women tend to decide very quickly when something's not working. Men don't. In every gym, there are those guys parading around with what they think is a six-pack. In reality, it's a beer belly screaming to be let out of the too-tight top. It's not attractive. Equally, we don't all need to see what religion you are—take your camel hoof home and go up a size in those silky short shorts.

THE GOT IT RIGHT-ERS

(Slow clap) Well done. You look perfectly equipped for the gym. You're probably all in black, with no muffin top anywhere, nothing straining, nothing unsightly falling out. Full marks.

THE OMGS

These are rarely seen, but it does happen:
- Men in vests with rainforest-hairy shoulders. Thick, horrible, NO.
- Women in transparent tights that they are either too old to wear, or that are being stretched to the max.
- Men wearing vests cut to the navel. Can these just be saved for your house maybe? We don't all want to see it. Show off.
- Men in short shorts. By all means wear them, but just watch out… the leg press can expose a lot more than you want to.

THE ROUTINERS

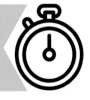

Want to know what it's like to be The Routiner? Then consider these analogies: you're in a boat and need to reach the other side of a lake, so you row and row, but only ever move a few feet, then stop. Or how about you spend your entire adult life on a diet, following strict instructions from a dietician, and lose a few pounds, but then the weight loss stagnates, despite your best efforts. Or maybe you're a hamster on "The Wheel." You spin, and spin, and spin, but get nowhere fast. Such is the life of The Routiner. For all intents and purposes, you're doing a great job of working out. You go the prescribed three times a week and only ever not turn up when you're seriously hungover. You take as gospel the plan set out for you by the personal trainer when you very first joined—you've been using it for two years now—which might be the very reason why you're no longer seeing results.

You're comfortable in your routine:

CARDIO	WEIGHTS
20 minutes' treadmill	10 x bicep curls (3 reps)
20 minutes' cross-trainer	10 x leg press (3 reps)
10 minutes' rowing machine	10 x deadlifts (3 reps)
STRETCH	REPEAT

Ask any personal trainer and they'll tell you this is... #basic. And the fact you've been peddling out this same routine time and time again is the exact reason why your body is no longer responding to it. Just like you eventually get immune to your favorite perfume or aftershave, your muscles start to get complacent. THIS IS BAD.

Some possible ideas to shake up your routine:
• Grab three protein shakes from the hands of body builders and juggle them while fast walking (or slow running) on the treadmill.
• Put on any Rihanna or Beyoncé track and cross-train to the beat. Your heart rate will soon increase. Don't lose it, though, you don't want to be that person to fall off backward.
• Spy a hottie across the gym floor, and midway through your row, jog over next to him/her and do 10 burpees. This'll definitely impress, maybe get you talking, and will shift extra pounds.

Socrates once said: "The secret of change is to focus all of your energy, not on fighting the old, but on building the new." So come on, it's time for a refresh of that old, dusty plan. New routine, new you. Trust the change, you'll no longer question why you slog away and reap none of the rewards. And not to scare you off completely, but if you're questioning yourself, there will be other gym-goers who have noticed too. #Judged.

THE PERSONAL TRAINERS

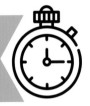

"My personal trainer told me that..." How many of you find yourself starting sentences like this now? Once upon a time it was "My therapist told me that..." but who needs to pay a shrink when your PT can do both things: coach you through a grueling workout and through life? Long gone are the days when a trainer's job was to "show you the ropes" when you join a gym. They're in it for the long haul. Two, three, four, five times a week—hell, some PTs end up marrying their clients just so they can see them less. And why is it that they always have the right thing to say to you when you need it the most? Clever little earners. Recognize any of these?

THE GBFT (AKA THE GAY BEST FRIEND TRAINER)

Easy to spot because of his hair-flicking and choreographed Rihanna workouts, this guy is the go-to for women who don't want to be a) judged by a fitter woman and b) can't handle a straight guy coming on to them for three hours a week. Besides anything, his clients always look like they're having the most fun—stretching with a length of marabou trim? YES, PLEASE!

THE EX-SQUADDIE

There's no time for fun with this one. The exact opposite of The GBFT, this PT is like a drill sergeant. Every single minute is accounted for, and when there's an awkward silence, he'll make you run on the spot. Having a water break is a luxury he doesn't like to grant, and don't even think about not finishing a set of press-ups! His mantra is simple and extremely cheesy— "No pain, no gain." Yeah, we haven't heard that one before!

THE BEEFCAKE

If it's gainz you want, this PT is for you. He doesn't look like he's wearing a comedy body-builder costume for nothing—it's all real. He has turned even the scrawniest people into bulging weight lifters, and prides himself on using everything in the gym as equipment—stand still for too long and he'll try to bench-press you. He has sachets of protein powder for each client after a session, whether you want it or not. It's the little things!

THE BIGGEST FAN

When you've had a crap day at work, the best release is to go and smash out a workout. Even better when your PT is feeding you lines of encouragement and congratulatory backslaps that you wish your boss was eager to dish out. Everything you do is "excellent" and "brilliant," and just when you thought you couldn't give one more punch, they use the "imagine it's your manager" line and you complete the set.

THE KNOW-IT-ALL

It's one thing paying for their expertise, but when it's forced on you unwillingly it becomes slightly annoying. You're quietly doing your own thing when you get a tap on the shoulder: "You're doing that all wrong!" Here's the thing… they might be right, they probably are, but that patronizing tone just makes you want to rugby tackle them to the ground.

THE NEW FRIEND

One minute they're coaching you through a new routine, the next you're in a bar with them doing shots. Don't worry, this isn't like a doctor-patient thing—no laws have been broken. It may feel odd to pay your buddy to work out with you, but without even knowing it they are changing your body for the good. Except when you wake up with a hangover. And here's you thinking you couldn't make any new friends after leaving school!

THE CREATIVE

Once upon a time, making up elaborate exercise routines was a job for personal trainers—that is, after all, what you pay them for. But since we all now think of ourselves as qualified fitness experts in our own right, nothing is off-limits when it comes to creative workouts. Clapping 10 times between fly lift reps to squatting with a barbell on your neck and kettlebells strapped to your belt, nothing is off-limits anymore. It's when you have to help someone down from the step machine because they've jammed it with a sweaty towel thinking that swinging it round their head, lasso-style, will tone the thighs and the triceps at once that you know it has gone one step (mind the pun) too far. If you are feeling creative, though, look no further... we've done the hard work for you and spoken to the experts (names withheld for fear of ridicule) to suggest some ingenious workouts to try, all based on routines they've witnessed... obviously!

ALL THE SINGLE LADIES
10 minutes on the step machine, 10 burpees, then the "Put a Ring On It" dance move. Repeat 10 times for Beyoncé-style thighs.

THE TRUMP
Blow up a life-size replica of The Donald and carry on as normal, using it as a punch bag.

THE ASSAULT COURSE

Using other gym-goers as markers, sprint as fast as you can to each person and back again—and you get extra points for knocking them over. After that, make your way from one end of the gym to the other, crawling under the handles of the treadmills and jumping over the bikes. Try this for as long as it takes before someone actually screams at you.

WORKOUT LOTTERY

Take a few pieces of paper and write a different exercise on each one (squats, running on the spot, push-ups, shaking your protein shake). Put them in a cup or holder, give them a shuffle, and take out five at random. There's your routine!

PARTNER UP

Get your other half, or whoever is nearest, to plank on the floor while you jump back and forth over them. Get them to slowly raise themselves up by leaning on their elbows until they are eventually in the Downward Dog pose, all the while you're jumping over them. The challenge is not to land directly on them.

BALLS

Using one of the big exercise balls, start at one end of the gym and roll yourself over and off the ball, then into five push-ups. Repeat all the way down the middle of the gym, taking no prisoners. If someone is in your way, see them as a threat and bulldoze over them.

ZUMBAWAY

Do one minute on the bike at full pelt, then quickly dismount and break into Zumba for one minute, or hula hoop if you have one spare (who has one spare?). Repeat 30 times. Although we reckon you would have had so many stares at this point, you'll just want to leave.

THE SOCIAL (STEP) CLIMBER

Washing the car, walking the dog, buying lunch, smashing your record number of minutes holding a plank... if you didn't put it on social media, it didn't happen. Narrating your entire day online is now considered as normal as swiping right to find a new love interest. If you're new to all this, here are some pointers to get you started on a social media workout extravaganza, observed in every single gym, anywhere:

Before getting out of the car, check yourself in on Facebook. Even if you go to the gym just because you like the café's soya flat whites, people will believe you actually did some exercise.

Just before you walk through the door, get up Snapchat, find the filter with the dog ears, and film yourself going in. Don't forget to tell your audience (of three, including your sister) that you're about "to smash the Granny out of the punching bag."

Take an obligatory selfie in the changing rooms showing off how there is literally not one other human in at 11.30pm on a Monday night. Wait for the "clapping hands" emoji from the people that are so unimpressed with you right now.

When you spot your gym crush, don't forget to tell Twitter how insane he/she looks and how much of a sweaty mess you are. Getting people to feel sorry for you because a) you're single and b) you're sad enough to be Tweeting about your gym crush is OK. But never share a picture of him/her... this is considered stalking, even by your standards.

Share a screen pic of your machine to prove to the world you burned exactly 769 calories. And don't forget a witty caption like, "Now I can have that Snickers!" (Yawn).

Taking a Boomerang of your legs opening and closing on the thigh adductor machine is standard practice, or get your buddy to take one of you doing sit-ups, but remember to take it from high above to avoid any stomach rolls or extra chins getting in shot. Filter as appropriate.

Post a time-lapse video on Insta of your 20-minute circuit routine. Don't expect many likes, though—it'll just make people feel bad about themselves because they can't be arsed and you can!

If you've got abs, show them off! A quick way to get thousands of likes and followers is to unleash the six-pack. Men, add a topless pic of you in a towel and you'll be an instant mini-celeb.

Posting a video looking in the mirror is all fun and games until people start to notice the hottie in the background. Then it's less about your workout and more about being a matchmaker.

Upload a "progress" shot, but make sure you're showing real results. We want washboard abs, firm pecs, toned legs... not a desperately sucked-in stomach and the "make me thinner" filter.

Do all the above three times a week and you'll be well on the way to becoming the gym social media star you dreamed of.

THE KIDS

Have you ever walked into the gym and thought you've accidentally stumbled into the local youth club? Terrifying, right? Teenagers out to impress each other are a frightening breed, and while a young Cruz Beckham is lambasted for working out in fear that his body growth will be stunted, parents all over the country are happy for their sprouts to head off for a workout. There are specific times this might occur: Sunday afternoons, during any school holiday, and during ASBO Hour—when all those, erm, slightly more troubled younger members of society should be at school but are, in fact, bunking to take their frustration out on a dumbbell or two. Youth gangs in the gym are viewed in the same light as a gaggle of old people—points for trying, but generally quite irritating to navigate round.

To watch is to learn: said group will usually consist of half boys, half girls, and, naturally, there will be a love triangle among them. Ultimately, though, they are all friends trying to figure out this thing called puberty, while occasionally doing a set of squat jumps. You'll notice some awkwardness between some of the boys and girls—the boys don't know where to look when the girls, half-covered with some kind of training bralette and skimpy leggings, attempt leg raises. It's as though they'd melt if they were to look them in the eye.

Attention spans are typically between 3–7 minutes, or until boredom kicks in or a Snapchat needs to be sent. A few pull-ups on the bar for the boys, some sit-ups for the girls, and then the whole gang will be off again over to the weights room where they'll no doubt get under the feet of a few burly body builders with no time for spotty little oiks. Their intention for joining might have been to get fit but, in reality, they're there for a social. Give them a shot of Sambuca and a cigarette, and they'd be much happier.

They crowd round a machine as though they are watching a fight in the school playground, and although most are actually probably kind-natured, you feel intimidated to go over to ask if they've finished so you can get on with the hard work. Strange really, isn't it? Their combined age probably adds up to yours, yet they act like a cackle of hyenas—relentless and imposing.

Group selfies on the rowing machines are common, sending pictures to a friend over the other side of the gym floor is de rigueur, and drawing attention to a new pair of Yeezys instead of working a single muscle group is #standard. All the while you're just left asking one question: why isn't there a "Yoof Hour," when they pump out Justin Bieber tunes and fake smoke, and provide selfie sticks instead of barbells?

THE BLINK AND YOU'LL MISS THEM JUNKIES →

We've all done it. Pulled ourselves up off the sofa, shoved on whatever clothes are nearest, and taken ourselves off to the gym, only to get there and lose all motivation. Gone. Disappeared. Just like that last gin and tonic the night before. You step onto a machine only to get off it a minute later. It's only natural, though, considering this is your fifth day in a row working out, but for some, this is what happens every. single. time.

You've spied this person on numerous occasions doing questionable routines that really leave them no fitter than if they'd stayed on the couch munching on a pack of Oreos. But instead of saying anything (because then you'd be considered The Know-It-All, page 35), you watch, intrigued. These people need to be studied, like David Attenborough analyzing why a sloth is incapable of moving at any great speed whatsoever…

In they walk, stopping at the mats to take a deep breath, as if to say, "Not this again." They put their headphones on and spend the next five minutes choosing something to listen to that might arouse some kind of drive. They warm up half-heartedly—a few neck rolls and a couple of lunges—and set off for the treadmills. (By this point you're on your fifth cycle program, one eye on the bike screen watching the calories burnt rack up, the other on The Sloth deciding between a stroll or a slow walk. You clock the minutes you've spent peddling—87—and get back to it.)

In the corner of your eye, you notice The Sloth demount the running machine like it's the hardest thing they've ever done before. You're on minute 90. Three minutes. Three whole minutes! You laugh to yourself as they make their way to the ab weights machine and attempt a set, but reach number six and give up. A glutton for punishment, they still haven't totally given up for some reason. They head to the rowing machine and let out a feeble 300 meters of quite frankly the limpest row you've ever seen.

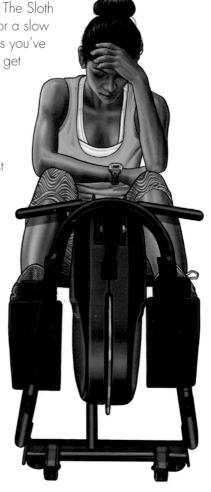

It isn't quite anger that you're feeling, it's more empathetic frustration. You know how they're feeling, but you want to just scream at them. And just before you actually do, they admit defeat, do half a hamstring stretch, and head home.

THE PREHISTORIC NOISE MAKERS

Anyone who frequents a gym will tell you that the number one most irritating person to work out next to is The Grunter. They can probably forgive Mr Body Builder—when you're lifting as much weight as a Mini Cooper, you expect a noise or too. But Mr Average? There's no excuse.

James is an Account Manager (whatever that means). Most days are pretty stressful for him, especially when the accounts he manages (again, whatever that means) include tricky clients. He also has a girlfriend he's not so sure about and who he gets annoyed with almost every time she speaks. His only release is at the gym, where you'll find him most evenings, when he is officially off the clock from managing his accounts (WTF?).

James likes to lift weights. He knows a personal trainer who once told him that you should only do 15 minutes' cardio to get your heart rate going, then hit the weights, hard. He now takes this as gospel. With his fast run done, he heads over to the free weights. James has very little muscle mass in his arms. He likes to think he does but, in reality, they resemble thin, slug-white sausages. He picks up his chosen dumbbells—usually the 12kgs, but sometimes the 14s if he has argued with the girlfriend he is about to dump. With one knee on the bench and the diagonal arm dangling over it with a weight in hand, he starts to pull it up toward his chest and back down. The first two up motions look easy, the rest get progressively harder. So much so, that he starts to sound like a cruise ship liner by the end of the set.

But he's not done. He goes in for another set. This time with an "URRRRGH" for every rep. Another level of Neanderthal. We're used to a Williams sister expelling these sounds when following through on a serve—Venus doesn't get to 129mph without a moan—but James? No. It's just not OK.

Suddenly the grunts turn into a hiss, then to a huff, then to a puffed-out cheek, then to what can only resemble some kind of sex noise. And just like that you're picturing James having sex, and this is what he sounds and looks like on orgasm. Again, that's just not OK.

When he's done, James puts back the weights, wipes his brow, walks over to the shoulder press machine, and starts the process all over again, blithely unaware that most of the people around him are staring and smirking.

Oh James!

THE CENTER OF ATTENTION

There's always one, in every single gym, anywhere in the world. That one person whose main purpose in life is to make it known that THEY are working out and that EVERYONE should know it. Fist pumps, exaggerated lunges, grunts not heard anywhere else in the wild. This gym-goer is so confident on the treadmill that he/she is most certainly making up for something else in their life: terrible job, annoying mother-in-law, relationship problems, the list is endless. Look around and notice how people will be smiling at them, not with them. Below are some classic traits of a true attention seeker; if you relate to these... #awkward.

THE MUSIC LOVER
You are so into the beat of this new track that not even the sight of your current crush will deter you from running that last mile. A hand in the air, whirling round and round to the song, is not uncommon. The occasional "whoop" might spur you on, but will send others over the edge. The only respite for other gym-goers is when the earphones fall out of your ears.

THE ENERGY FEELER
After five reps of 12 burpees, "normal" people would collapse in a pool of sweat on the floor. You, however, jump up and sling a barbell behind your head. After eight hours at work and one too many emails from the boss, "normal" people just need 20 minutes on the cross-trainer, but you're on 69 minutes and show no signs of giving up.

THE BALL SMASHER

We are, of course, referring to medicine balls (or ball weights). You know The Center of Attention is working out as soon as you walk through the doors, thanks to the resounding smash of heavy leather globes dropping to the floor. Even through vintage Sugababes, you can hear the grunt, followed by the thump, over and over again. Yes, we know that's the point of the balls, but when you're purple in the face, it might be time to stop. This person does not.

THE PROTEIN SHAKER

You haven't even finished putting down the weights before you start vigorously shaking that plastic bottle. You guzzle the pink gloop down as if you've never had a drink before, while the rest of us just wish it was a gin and tonic.

THE LOOK

You take color blocking as a challenge, not a trend. Whoever told you that an orange racer-back top and red and pink striped leggings are OK is no friend. And those new ombre shorts-over-meggings (man leggings) that you now sport thanks to some low-rent reality TV star are, erm, statement.

THE MAN IN THE MIRROR

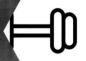

This isn't an ode to Michael Jackson. This is an ode to those men—practically every man—in the gym whose best friend is the mirror. They're in a deep, passionate, long-term relationship with each other. They can't, as much as they try, live without each other.

This is how the romantic story goes: it happened, well, the first time he ever went to the gym. There he was, pounding the cardio, minding his own business, when suddenly their eyes met. They couldn't stop staring at each other. Instant infatuation. For a full five minutes they just stood still, opposite each other, gazing deeply and intensely. The tension was palpable. There was instant chemistry, a spark so cosmic that everyone around them noticed it too. (It was, in fact, his iPhone flash reflection.) It truly was love at first sight. Every subsequent time they bumped into each other their love grew more deeply, their admiration more passionately, their adoration more vehemently. When they were apart in the gym, they pined for each other, they longed to see one another. They were happier when they were face to face, staring longingly, just like that first meeting. And they lived happily ever after.

That's the Cinderella version. In reality, what we have is a man so vain, so into himself that he can't do three lat pulldowns without checking in with his reflection to make sure his perfectly coiffed hair is still in place. It must be so exhausting, all that preening and grooming while simultaneously trying to do a workout. And the only person he's trying to impress is… himself! Narcissus would be so proud—he has mini protégés all round the globe keeping his legacy alive and well.

But the ones that are truly exasperating, the men (don't think for a minute we're being sexist… there are far more male gym narcissists than women) who really do give a new meaning to the word vain, are those who pull up their tops to reveal (most of the time) a full set of (strained) abs, just to check they are still there, in case they suddenly dropped off. And those who do a set of 12 bicep curls, then flash their guns at themselves in the mirror, as if their reflection is about to pipe up and congratulate them. Do these men not realize us "normal" folk are looking at them and laughing, like we are watching a real-life, live sketch show? Silly question really. It's pure comedy, though.

How about a social experiment? A nominated gym should fit two-way mirrors all round it, Big Brother-style, with body language experts studying these vain animals. Filmed and edited together, this screams of the next new hit reality show that charts just how far narcissists will go. Keeping Up with The Narcissists maybe?

THE HEAVY SWEATERS

The risk of doing anything in a public space is that you open yourself up to being looked at, judged, ridiculed even. Take, for instance, falling asleep on an aeroplane. Who hasn't stared at that person with their face pressed up against the window, snoring and dribbling all at the same time? Similarly at the gym, if you tend to perspire an abnormal amount, expect people to look at you.

We are all human, we all get hot, we all sweat. In fact, when you're sprinting up a hill on the treadmill or about to take off on the spin bike, you want to sweat. As soon as you break out, you know you are actually doing something, it's working, you're burning calories and fat. But there are those unfortunate souls that suffer from what some (no one in particular) like to call HSS—Heavy Sweating Syndrome.

Two minutes on the machine and you're dripping. Another five and you're pouring. Give it 10 and it's like The *Poseidon Adventure*. If you had a plug, this is the time you'd want to stuff it with something. But you just can't. The more you move, the more sweat your body produces. You grab six towels on your way in, one for each piece of equipment you come in contact with, such is your excretion problem. Short of walking round with a bucket permanently underneath you, the only way to deal with the Sweat Situation is with more and more towels. Soon, they'll start to charge you for dry-cleaning.

There are those *awful* people, though, those that may not be particularly heavy sweaters but still let out a fair amount, who don't wipe up after themselves at all. You'll never see them with a courtesy bit of tissue. They'll be finished on the rowing machine and the seat will have a wet imprint of their backside, or their time on the treadmill will be up and the belt will be soaked. You get on it, and slip over, cursing their horrid, unhygienic attitude.

The worst of the worst, though, happens just when your workout is over: you're half dead, you want to go home to have your protein-rich dinner, but you need to stretch for just five minutes to cool down. You spot a free mat, head over to it, get on all fours, and roll over onto your back. You put your head down to rest it for a minute, only to make direct contact between your neck and a cold, rancid pool of someone else's sweat. You quickly sit up, swear until you feel calm, and wipe the back of your head and the mat, storming off in the process. If you know, you know.

And people wonder why the gym sometimes smells like a secondhand clothes store in the middle of the Sahara Desert!

THE HIPSTER

The irony of spotting a hipster at the gym is that they are supposed to be dead against anything mainstream. Their cult status means they try to stay outside of society's norms; they do all they can to be "different." But it's all catching up with them. Nostalgia is so in right now, and you're no one if you're not wearing something that was previously owned by a tree-hugging, tree-smoking person from the '60s. Though they may like to think they go under that radar, there are clear signs The Hipster is among you on your daily workout:

CLOTHING

A stretchy training top is the enemy of The Hipster. They can only do a workout in a top if it:

    a) has a nearly worn band logo or slogan with at least one expletive

    b) has a scoop neck or no neck at all

    c) has a panel of dirty mesh somewhere

    d) is a shirt and braces combo

    e) is a vest that shows off a thick layer of shoulder and chest hair (him and possibly her).

On the bottoms, expect either Richard Simmons-esque short shorts, exposing uber pale legs, or super-skinny leggings. The only accessory is a sweatband, worn over long hair so that it holds it down, rather than away from the face. The main prerequisite, though, of any clothing is that it is at least 20 years old so that you can call it vintage and actually mean it. Keep clear of a sweaty Hipster, though… the smell of dusty old fabric will make even the strongest stomach heave.

HAIR

You'll know a Hipster is working out next to you by that strangely familiar scent of unwashed hair. You know, that sweetly stale smell that you try to mask with dry shampoo, but The Hipster embraces as a sign of their rebellion. Usually he has shoulder-length locks and a beard to match, like some kind of form out of Disney's *Fantasia*, and she has colored hair with a side fringe that starts at the top of her ear.

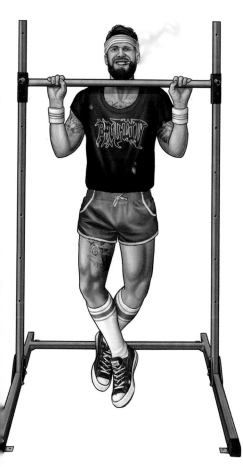

FOOTWEAR

Forget brand-new Nike or Adidas kicks. Oh no. The Hipster is more of a fan of nearly dead Converse, so battered and worn that you could send them to a Third World country and they'd send them back saying they aren't that desperate. The Hipster will attempt to work out in a canvas shoe, but soon realize they're defeated when the sole literally falls off after a light jog. There are those that take it to the absolute extreme though—BARE. FOOT. The risk of Athlete's Foot alone is enough to stop writing this.

TATTOOS

Although it's common now for even the most un-hipster of us to have tattoos, it's The Hipster who likes to show theirs off at the gym. And it's not just one or two... full sleeves, all-over backs, even some on the face. Catch them in the changing room, and you might even spot an inked "MOM" circling a nipple, a yin and yang sign over a belly button, or a mustache in an area you didn't think it possible to tattoo.

CIGARETTE BREAKS

Smoking for hipsters is like lying for politicians—they go hand in hand. Literally. And just because they aren't in a dive bar with peanut shells strewn across the floor and strange rock playing, doesn't mean they won't light up. If there wasn't a smoking ban inside, they'd puff away on the bikes, but watch them quite happily finish a round of weights, roll up, and head outside. Only to come back in and carry on as normal.

THE BULLSH***ERS

You have to watch what you say these days, everywhere. They say you're always two feet away from someone who is happy to post all-things #overheard on their Twitter account. The more ridiculous the statement, the more likes and retweets it gets. The gym is a breeding ground for big egos, big muscles, and big statements. But what do they really mean?

I've got to do an extra half an hour of cardio today... I had a pizza for lunch!
And a glass of wine before the pizza, a dessert after, and a family-size bar of chocolate before bed.

No pain, no gainz.
Suffer in silence or else everyone will think you're a big wuss.

The men's changing room has better lighting for selfies.
I like to take selfies and make sure I get the fat old naked man in the background to send to the "boys" Whatsapp group.

Leg day!
I convince myself that my calves are getting stronger and bigger, but in reality they resemble Twiglets.

I haven't been for a while because I've had an injury.
I haven't been for a while because quite frankly I couldn't be arsed and had better things to do, like, erm, have a life.

I hate it when people say I look like a body builder!
I love it when people say I look like a body builder. It makes me feel like Arnold Schwarzenegger. It makes me feel really big and strong. Like a "real" man.

Quality not quantity.
I can get away with doing way less than I have to.

The squat rack is for squats, not curls bro!
Get off this thing and let my ego grow a tiny bit more while I show you how it's really done!

I love to work out, but I hate sweating.
I'm so lazy, all I want to do is sit on the power plate and play Candy Crush.

If you don't feel like you've been hit by a bus, you haven't done legs day properly.
Honestly, I'd rather a bus hit me than have to do legs day again.

THE CARDIO FREAKS

You'll soon spot The Cardio Freaks. They hit those machines hard. But it's OK. They don't mind. They love cardio. They haven't actually picked up a weight in a decade—they use only their own body weight as resistance. On the rear window of their car, tucked away in the bottom left-hand corner, is a bright pink sticker that reads: CARDIO IS MY RELIGION. These people are devout.

Like The Cardio Freak you might also have good reason to never go near the weights room:

- The feeling of pure dread when you pick up a weight and immediately know that you can't lift it, but you need to style it out, so you try—only to drop it on your big toe.
- Intimidation from the beefy meatheads that are all puffing and panting their way through hundreds of reps, with bulging biceps, rippling stomachs, and tree-trunk thighs.
- The force field of endorphins and testosterone that prevents you from entering, like an electrified fence.

So, being forced to keep away from the weights, they nail the cardio instead. Their routine goes something like this:

1. Stretch
2. Cross-trainer for 40 minutes
3. Treadmill for 30 minutes
4. Bathroom break
5. Rowing machine for 20 minutes
6. Spinning class for 50 minutes

You see The Cardio Freaks at the end of their session and they look broken. Bright red faces, pouring with sweat. They look like little punctured lilos, but yet they come back day after day, week after week. Their heart rates must be fantastic, sure, and they can probably eat exactly what they like at any time of the day, but they have such little muscle mass that even if they did attempt a round of weights, they're likely to snap a limb or two. "Leg day" (see page 55) would be an absolute disaster for them.

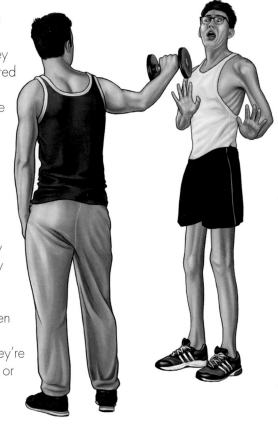

The little laminated signs stuck to each machine that asks if everyone can keep their time to 15 minutes in busy periods are completely ignored by The Cardio Freak. They see that as a challenge, not a request, much to the chagrin of their fellow gym buddies. These are also the people that book into cardio classes the second the next week's times are released. Woe betide anyone that stands in the way of them and a bike at spin class.

THE LUNCHTIME JUNKIE

With a gym space popping up on every street corner now, rivaling doggy day care and Starbucks, it makes it easy to access one at any time of the day. Early morning opening times for the really eager ones, 24-hour gyms for those with no other time to work out than 2am, some that open up especially for you, whenever you want (if you're an A-lister, obvs), but all have one thing in common. Come midday, they will be heaving with men and women ready to rip off their work suits and have a short, sharp burst of energy-filled workout time before having to head back to the office.

It's now deemed acceptable to skip actually having lunch on your lunch break and replace it with an express spin or Legs, Bums, and Tums class, or for the lifters among us, 45 minutes of chest/arms/back/shoulders/legs (delete as appropriate). Bosses across the world have now turned a blind eye to their staff doing a quick Superman-style change into their short shorts. In fact, it's often the managers managing their lunchtime sessions too.

You can now get away with suggesting that going to the gym halfway through the work day is "good for my soul"/ "will help my creative juices to flow"/ "will make me happier and therefore give me better job satisfaction." One thing is for sure, HR would have a hard time to intervene with this one. They ain't got a leg to stand on, so to speak.

It's obvious who are the workers working out though… upping the incline on the treadmill while simultaneously negotiating eating a sandwich, rowing furiously while screaming down the phone at an assistant to get their post-lunch meeting to wait in reception, and updating a spreadsheet in between doing a set of curls. It should be an escape from the office, not a time to bore others with work politics. But alas, the majority of people at the gym at lunchtime are probably all in the same boat.

If it shows one skill though, it's excellent time-keeping (you can add that to your resumé). Typically, it's 37 minutes' exercising, three stretching, three going to the bathroom after holding it in all morning because you simply cannot do a Number Two at work, seven to shower, dry yourself using the hairdryer, and get dressed, and 10 to get back to your desk. Well done you!

There is often talk of doing office workouts, but a yoga session in the board room or a HIIT (high-intensity interval training) class in the canteen isn't as appealing as plugging your headphones in and stepping away from your emails for that precious hour. Besides anything, you really don't want to see overweight Sandra from accounts in her leotard, thank you very much.

THE LINES LEARNER

Mostly found in capital cities or towns that support Local Theater, this gym-goer might also be known as The Out of Work Actor. Have you ever spotted Nicole Kidman on a rowing machine, or Tom Hanks finishing off his chest presses with script in hand? Didn't think so. This person has vetoed the local coffee shop, park, church, or their own bedroom and has instead chosen to memorize their lines in the gym. If you thought it was a skill to learn 250 pages of pure monologue, consider perfecting the holding-script-swinging-kettlebell dance. There are ways you can identify the type of actor, too:

THE BLOCKBUSTER STAR

Showing a range of emotions, from ecstasy to deep depression, in a matter of minutes, while simultaneously negotiating the cross-trainer. You might see her pointing a fake gun at the person next to her in a spin class, or faking an orgasm in the midst of a steep incline. Some have even witnessed him/her rehearsing an Oscar-winning speech. You've gotta admire the ambition.

THE TV ACTOR

Because of the short amount of time between receiving a script and actually filming a soap, this actor is often seen laughing to themselves on the treadmill or crying while stretching. But these are all real emotions. Not acted. Their character has either told the best joke, or has just been killed off. Either way, it's easy to spot a TV actor: they'll be the ones happily signing autographs and taking selfies. All press is good press.

THE MUSICAL PERFORMER

They didn't learn Bob Fosse jazz hands in vain. Learning dance routines is just as common as learning lines to a big Broadway number. The treadmill is the perfect machine to practice something from *Chicago*, while the very top of the step machine is ideal training for that balcony scene in *Evita*. Some people sing the occasional word or two of a Beyoncé or Justin Bieber song, but you guessed it... the musical theater actor blasts out a full eight bars of *I Dreamed a Dream* with a 20-pound weight hanging off the end of their foot.

REALITY

If you think reality shows are not scripted, just rip the wad of paper from the hands of someone who looks like they could be a Kardashian or are a Real Housewife from Chelsea. You'll soon see that the passionate, loving moment or raging argument is repeated line for line, parrot fashion. If you want to know what happens between those two, just make sure to sidle up to the reality TV star, mid-row, and take your earphones out. Thank us later.

And remember, if you do spot an actor during your workout, there are plenty of magazines who would pay decent money for a #Spotted shot!

THE FREE PASSES

While being a "Coupon Queen" once meant you are overly frugal, now it's a way of life for most people. Everyone is doing it. Who doesn't like to save a bit when they can? Those BOGOF offers sell themselves. There are even apps now that let you know when your favorite shops and online stores have money-off vouchers, which makes you think the people coming up with said apps must be the most money-conscious of everyone. There's nothing quite like getting a free pass for the gym though, is there?

You're that person who'll walk through a train station and take all the handouts from those pushy out-of-work-actors trying to market a brand—mini cans of a new soft drink, a sample size bar of chocolate, some new brand of energy 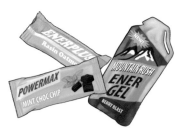 gels and power bars, a goody bag that you find is just full of press releases, but it was FREE so who cares! And, of course, the two-week trial cards from the (on purpose) incredibly cute personal trainers.

You spend no time deliberating whether you'll use it or not, you've been threatening to join a gym, well, forever, and these passes are like gold dust, so you jump at the chance. Literally. You're straight there and on a cardio machine.

You work out that in two weeks you could substantially tone your left bicep, and then find another gym promotion to do the right. Or if it's fat burning you prefer, you've totted up that you stand to obliterate nearly 10,000 calories in 14 days. Time is precious, so you clear your diary.

Oh no! You've suddenly turned into that person who on an all-inclusive vacation, is the one calculating how many gin and tonics they can fit into the 16 hours of being awake. But who actually cares? You're here to work out, and that's exactly what you're doing. You take full advantage. Whereas your contemporaries who actually pay to be there are in and out in an hour, you take your time. Your workout might take you a couple of hours after you try (and fail) a round on every single machine. Then you'll go and make full use of the sauna and steam room, leaving just before you actually cook yourself, and finally take a long, luxurious shower, pumping the shower gel attached to the wall into your own empty bottle because, well, it's free!

But regular gym-goers worry not. The Coupon Queen/King won't be sticking around for long. God forbid they pay for an actual membership. No, they'll be there every day for two weeks solid, and then you won't see them again. Not until the gym is desperate for membership sign-ups again. They will, however, hop from one gym to another giving free trials, and before they know it, they've had a full 52 weeks for FREE. God loves a trier!

INDEX